WALL PILATES WORKOUTS FOR WOMEN

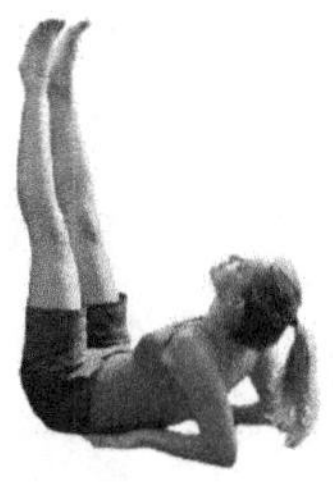

Sculpting Strength and Flexibility with Wall Pilates Workouts for Women

By
Larissa Booth

TABLE OF CONTENTS

INTRODUCTION

Brief overview of Wall Pilates

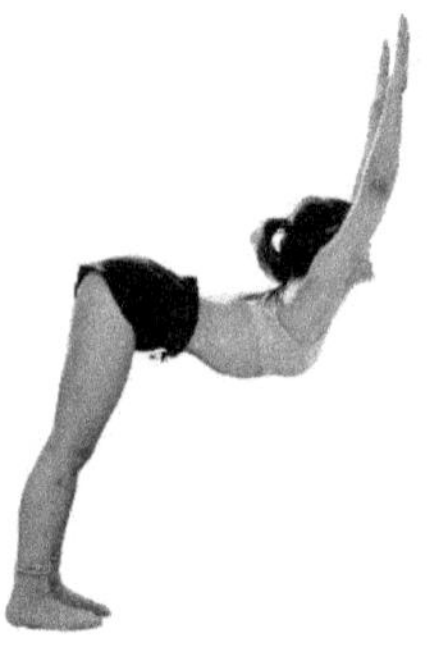

Welcome to the invigorating world of Wall Pilates, a fitness journey designed to elevate not just your physical strength but also your overall well-being. In the upcoming chapters, we'll explore how this innovative approach to Pilates can bring about transformative changes, especially tailored for the needs of women.

Wall Pilates is a dynamic exercise method that incorporates the support of a wall to enhance traditional Pilates movements. It's about finding stability, improving posture, and building a strong foundation from the ground up. Whether you're a beginner or already familiar with Pilates, the wall becomes your ally in sculpting a leaner, more toned physique.

As we delve deeper, you'll discover the unique advantages Wall Pilates offers, blending the core principles of Pilates with the added benefit of wall support. Get ready to embrace a workout routine that not only challenges your body but also empowers you on your fitness journey.

Benefits specific to women's fitness

Now, let's explore the tailored benefits that Wall Pilates brings to women's fitness. Beyond the conventional advantages of Pilates, this approach is finely tuned to address the specific needs and goals of women.

One notable benefit lies in core strengthening, essential for maintaining a strong and supportive center. Wall Pilates engages key muscles, including the core, pelvic floor, and hips, contributing to improved stability and posture. For women, this can be particularly beneficial in addressing common concerns such as postpartum recovery and pelvic floor health.

Additionally, Wall Pilates offers a targeted approach to toning the upper and lower body. With exercises like wall push-ups and leg lifts, you'll sculpt lean muscles, enhancing both strength and flexibility. These movements are crafted to align with the natural biomechanics of a woman's body, fostering a balanced and functional fitness routine.

As we progress, we'll uncover how Wall Pilates uniquely caters to women's fitness needs, providing a holistic approach that goes beyond the physical benefits, delving into mindfulness and overall well-being. Get ready to embrace a workout routine designed with your specific goals in mind.

Importance of proper form and safety

Now, let's emphasize the crucial foundation of Wall Pilates: proper form and safety. In the world of fitness, it's not just about the workout; it's about how you do it.

Maintaining correct form during Wall Pilates exercises is paramount to maximize effectiveness and prevent injuries. The support of the wall adds a dimension of stability, but it's essential to align your body correctly to ensure targeted muscle engagement. This focus on precision not only enhances the workout's impact but also minimizes the risk of strain or discomfort.

Safety is at the forefront of Wall Pilates, making it an accessible and sustainable option for women of all fitness levels. The controlled movements, coupled with the support from the wall, create an environment where you can challenge yourself without compromising your well-being. This emphasis on safety makes Wall Pilates an ideal choice for those navigating fitness journeys, ensuring a positive and injury-free experience.

As we continue our exploration, keep in mind the importance of prioritizing form and safety. It's not just about completing the exercises; it's about doing them right, fostering a workout routine that is both effective and sustainable in the long run.

CHAPTER 1

Getting Started

Basics of Pilates principles

Let's kick off your Wall Pilates journey by laying down the fundamentals – the basics of Pilates principles. Understanding these principles sets the stage for a successful and effective workout.

First and foremost is the principle of centering. Pilates is all about building strength from your core, the powerhouse of your body. Wall Pilates takes this a step further by using the support of the wall to enhance your connection to your center, ensuring each movement originates from a stable core.

Next up is concentration. In the world of Wall Pilates, it's not about going through the motions; it's about mindful movement. Concentrating on your body's alignment, muscle engagement, and breathing patterns amplifies the impact of each exercise, promoting both physical and mental well-being.

Control is another key principle. Wall Pilates encourages deliberate, controlled movements. The wall provides support, but it's your controlled actions that truly activate and sculpt your muscles. This emphasis on control not only refines your movements but also reduces the risk of strain.

Precision is the fourth principle, emphasizing the importance of accuracy in each movement. Wall Pilates encourages you to be aware of your body's positioning, ensuring that every exercise targets the intended muscle groups. This precision elevates the effectiveness of your workout, bringing you closer to your fitness goals.

Lastly, let's talk about flow. In Wall Pilates, seamless transitions between exercises are essential. The fluidity of movement not only enhances the overall experience but also promotes grace and efficiency in your workout routine.

So, as you embark on your Wall Pilates journey, keep these principles in mind – centering, concentration, control, precision, and flow. They're the compass guiding you toward a fulfilling and effective fitness routine.

Necessary equipment and setup

Now, let's delve into the practical aspects of starting your Wall Pilates workouts – the necessary equipment and setup. The beauty of Wall Pilates lies in its simplicity, requiring minimal gear for a rewarding exercise experience.

First and foremost, you'll need a sturdy and flat wall. Choose a space where you have enough room to extend your limbs comfortably. Make sure the wall is free of obstructions, providing a secure backdrop for your exercises.

For added comfort, a Pilates mat or a non-slip yoga mat is beneficial, especially if your workout involves floor exercises. This ensures a cushioned surface and prevents slipping during movements.

Incorporate a small prop like a Pilates ball or resistance band for variety and added challenge in certain exercises. These affordable and accessible tools can elevate your workout intensity and engage different muscle groups.

As for attire, opt for comfortable and breathable workout wear. The goal is to move freely without restriction, allowing you to fully immerse yourself in the exercises.

Now, with your wall, mat, and optional props in place, you're ready to start your Wall Pilates journey. The simplicity of the setup ensures that you can seamlessly integrate these workouts into your daily routine, making fitness a convenient and enjoyable part of your lifestyle. So, find your wall, lay down your mat, and let's get started on the path to a stronger, more empowered you.

Warm-up routines tailored for women

Before diving into the invigorating world of Wall Pilates, it's crucial to lay the foundation with a warm-up specifically tailored for women. This not only primes your body for the upcoming exercises but also minimizes the risk of injury and ensures a more effective workout.

Start with gentle neck rotations and shoulder rolls to release tension. Incorporate hip circles to promote flexibility in the pelvic region, which is particularly beneficial for women's overall well-being.

Move on to dynamic stretches, such as leg swings and arm circles, to increase blood flow to major muscle groups. These movements prepare your body for the upcoming Wall Pilates exercises, gradually elevating your heart rate.

Focus on core activation with pelvic tilts and gentle twists. Engaging your core in the warm-up primes those essential muscles for the targeted work they'll receive during Wall Pilates, promoting better stability and control.

As a woman, paying attention to your pelvic floor is key. Include Kegel exercises in your warm-up to strengthen this area, contributing to improved bladder control and pelvic health.

Finish the warm-up with controlled breathing exercises. Deep, rhythmic breaths not only oxygenate your muscles but also center your mind, setting a positive tone for the Wall Pilates session ahead.

Remember, the warm-up isn't just a formality – it's a crucial step in ensuring a safe and effective workout. Take the time to gradually prepare your body for the movements to come, and you'll find yourself better equipped to reap the full benefits of Wall Pilates. Now, with your body primed and ready, let's embark on this transformative fitness journey together.

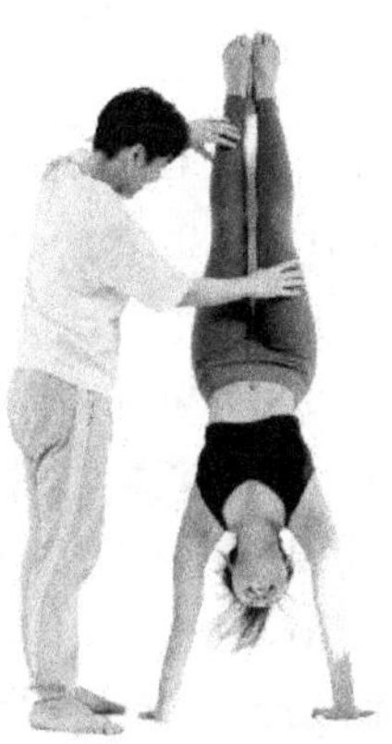

CHAPTER 2

Wall Pilates Exercises

Core strengthening

Now, let's delve into the heart of Wall Pilates – core strengthening exercises. This fundamental aspect not only builds a robust core but also forms the cornerstone of your entire fitness journey.

Begin with pelvic tilts against the wall. This simple yet effective movement engages your lower abdominal muscles, enhancing core stability. The wall provides support, allowing you to focus on controlled movements and proper muscle activation.

Next, explore leg raises with wall support. This exercise targets both the lower abdominal and hip flexor muscles, promoting a balanced and sculpted core. The wall serves as a guide, ensuring your movements are precise and controlled.

Transition into plank variations using the wall. Whether it's a traditional plank, side plank, or forearm plank, the wall adds an extra dimension to these exercises. This engages not only your core but also your shoulders and back muscles, contributing to overall upper body strength.

These core-strengthening exercises lay the groundwork for improved posture, enhanced stability, and a toned midsection. As you progress through these movements, pay attention to the connection between your breath and each contraction, fostering a mind-body synergy that defines the essence of Wall Pilates.

So, with your back against the wall and determination in your core, let's embark on this journey to fortify the center of your strength and vitality. The wall is your ally, supporting you in sculpting a resilient and empowered core.

Let's break down these core-strengthening Wall Pilates exercises to guide you through each movement.

Pelvic Tilts Against the Wall:
Begin by standing with your back against the wall, feet hip-width apart. Inhale as you tilt your pelvis towards the wall, engaging your lower abs. Exhale as you return to the neutral position. The wall provides support, ensuring your movements are controlled. Aim for 15-20 repetitions, gradually increasing as your core strength improves.

Leg Raises with Wall Support:

Lie on your back with the wall at your side. Place your hands under your hips for added support. Inhale as you lift your legs towards the wall, engaging your lower abs. Exhale as you lower them back down. The wall guides your leg movement, promoting proper form. Start with 10-12 repetitions, gradually progressing as your strength develops.

Plank Variations:
For the traditional plank, position yourself facing the wall in a push-up position, arms extended. Maintain a straight line from head to heels, engaging your core. Hold for 30 seconds to a minute, gradually extending the duration as you build strength.

For side planks, position yourself sideways with one forearm on the wall. Lift your hips, forming a straight line from head to heels. Hold for 20-30 seconds on each side. The wall provides stability, allowing you to focus on the targeted muscles.

These exercises, when performed with consistency and attention to form, contribute to a resilient and toned core. Let the wall be your guide, supporting you in every controlled movement as you build the foundation of a stronger and more empowered you.

Upper body toning

Let's now shift our focus to upper body toning exercises in the realm of Wall Pilates.

Wall Push-ups:
Stand facing the wall, arms extended at shoulder height. Inhale as you lean towards the wall, bending your elbows. Exhale as you push back to the starting position. The wall provides a supportive surface, making this a beginner-friendly yet effective exercise. Aim for 15-20 repetitions, gradually increasing as your upper body strength improves.

Shoulder Blade Squeezes:
Stand with your back against the wall, feet hip-width apart. Inhale as you squeeze your shoulder blades together, focusing on the muscles between your shoulder blades. Exhale as you release. The wall acts as a reference point, ensuring proper alignment. Perform 12-15 repetitions, feeling the engagement in your upper back.

Tricep Dips Using the Wall:
Sit on the floor with your back against the wall, palms on the wall behind you. Inhale as you lift your hips, bending your elbows to lower your body towards the floor. Exhale as you push back up. The wall supports your back, allowing for controlled

tricep engagement. Start with 10-12 repetitions, gradually increasing as your tricep strength develops.

These upper body toning exercises, when integrated into your Wall Pilates routine, target key muscles in your arms, shoulders, and upper back. The wall serves as a dependable partner, ensuring proper form and support throughout each movement. As you embrace these exercises, feel the transformation in your upper body strength and the confidence it brings to your overall fitness journey.

Lower body sculpting

Let's dive into the world of lower body sculpting with these targeted Wall Pilates exercises.

Wall Sits with Variations:
Position yourself with your back against the wall and lower into a seated position, as if sitting in an imaginary chair. The wall provides support as you hold this position, engaging your quads and glutes. To add variation, incorporate small pulses or lift one leg at a time. Aim for 30 seconds to a minute in the wall sit, gradually increasing duration as your lower body strength improves.

Leg Lifts and Circles:

Lie on your side with the wall at your back for stability. Inhale as you lift your top leg towards the wall, engaging your outer thigh. Exhale as you lower it down. For circles, lift the leg and make controlled circular motions, targeting both inner and outer thighs. Repeat on each side for 12-15 repetitions, feeling the burn in your lower body.

Inner Thigh Exercises Against the Wall:
Lie on your back with your feet against the wall, forming a 90-degree angle at your hips and knees. Inhale as you open your legs, engaging your inner thighs. Exhale as you bring them back together. The wall supports your legs, allowing for precise movements. Aim for 15-20 repetitions, gradually increasing as your inner thigh strength develops.

These lower body sculpting exercises, complemented by the support of the wall, work towards toning and strengthening key muscle groups. The controlled movements bring awareness to your lower body, fostering both physical and mental well-being. Embrace the burn, let the wall be your ally, and feel the empowerment as you sculpt and define your lower body through Wall Pilates.

CHAPTER 3

Advanced Wall Pilates

Incorporating props for added challenge

As you progress on your Wall Pilates journey, let's explore the realm of advanced exercises by incorporating props. These additions bring a heightened challenge to your routine, taking your strength and flexibility to new levels.

Pilates Ball:
Integrate a Pilates ball to intensify core workouts. For example, during pelvic tilts against the wall, place the ball between your knees. Squeeze the ball as you tilt your pelvis, adding resistance and engaging additional muscles. This challenges your stability and deepens the impact on your core. Aim for 15-20 repetitions, gradually increasing as your strength builds.

Resistance Band:
Enhance leg exercises with a resistance band. During leg lifts with wall support, place the band around your ankles. The resistance adds tension, intensifying the workout for your outer thighs and

glutes. Perform 12-15 repetitions on each leg, feeling the burn and gradual progression in strength.

Hand Weights:

Incorporate hand weights for upper body toning. During wall push-ups, hold weights in each hand. This adds resistance to your arm movements, targeting your chest, shoulders, and triceps more intensely. Start with lighter weights and aim for 12-15 repetitions, gradually increasing as your upper body strength advances.

Intensifying core exercises

Now, let's delve into advanced techniques for intensifying core exercises in your Wall Pilates routine. These modifications will not only challenge your core muscles more effectively but also elevate the overall impact of your workout.

Elevated Leg Raises:

During leg raises with wall support, take it up a notch by incorporating an elevated surface. Place a sturdy bench or step under your feet, maintaining contact with the wall. This increases the range of motion, engaging your lower abs and hip flexors more intensely. Aim for 10-12 repetitions, gradually progressing as your core strength improves.

Twisting Planks:

Advance your plank variations by adding a twist. In a traditional plank against the wall, rotate your torso to bring one knee towards your chest. Alternate sides, engaging your obliques and deep core muscles. The wall ensures stability, allowing you to focus on controlled twists. Perform 15-20 rotations on each side, feeling the dynamic engagement in your core.

Hollow Body Holds:
Lie on your back with your legs extended against the wall and arms reaching overhead. Lift your legs and upper body off the ground, creating a "hollow" position. This challenges your entire core, especially the lower abs. Hold for 20-30 seconds, gradually increasing the duration as you build strength.

By incorporating these advanced techniques, you'll intensify the focus on your core muscles, fostering a deeper connection and enhanced results. The wall remains your reliable support, allowing you to push your limits and experience the transformative power of advanced core exercises in the realm of Wall Pilates.

Progressive routines for continuous improvement

To ensure continuous improvement in your Wall Pilates journey, let's explore the concept of progressive routines. These structured plans gradually challenge your body, fostering strength, flexibility, and overall fitness development over time.

Week 1-2: Foundation Building
Focus on mastering the basics. Emphasize proper form in exercises like pelvic tilts, wall push-ups, and leg lifts. Keep repetitions moderate and focus on building a strong foundation for future progress.

Week 3-4: Introducing Variations
Incorporate variations of exercises you've mastered. Add twists to your plank variations, try different leg lift angles, and explore diverse ways to engage your core. This introduces variety while still emphasizing control and form.

Week 5-6: Adding Props
Integrate props like a Pilates ball or resistance band for added resistance. Experiment with these during core, upper, and lower body exercises. The added challenge helps target specific muscle groups and enhances overall strength.

Week 7-8: Advanced Techniques

Gradually introduce advanced techniques discussed earlier, such as elevated leg raises, twisting planks, and hollow body holds. Focus on quality over quantity, ensuring controlled movements to maximize effectiveness.

Week 9-10: Full-Body Integration

Combine exercises into seamless routines, targeting both upper and lower body in a single session. Emphasize fluid transitions between movements, enhancing coordination and overall body awareness.

Week 11-12: Intensity Boost

Increase the intensity of your workouts by adding more repetitions, longer hold times, or reducing rest between exercises. This final phase challenges your endurance and allows you to witness the cumulative improvements in strength and stamina.

Remember, progression is about consistency and incremental adjustments. Listen to your body, celebrate small victories, and gradually push your boundaries. The wall remains a constant support, guiding you through each phase of your progressive Wall Pilates routines, ensuring a continuous and fulfilling fitness journey.

CHAPTER 4

Targeting Specific Concerns

Posture correction exercises

Now, let's address a common concern with targeted Wall Pilates exercises – posture correction. These movements are designed to strengthen key muscle groups, promoting better alignment and overall posture.

Shoulder Blade Retractions:
Stand with your back against the wall, arms extended at shoulder height. Inhale as you squeeze your shoulder blades together, focusing on the muscles between them. Exhale as you release. This exercise reinforces proper upper back alignment, countering the effects of slouching.

Wall Angels:
Lie on your back with your entire spine against the wall. Extend your arms overhead, palms facing the wall. Slowly slide your arms down while keeping them in contact with the wall. This movement engages your back muscles, opening up the chest and contributing to improved posture.

Wall Supported Back Extension:

Stand facing the wall with your hands on it at shoulder height. Inhale as you arch your back, lifting your chest towards the ceiling. Exhale as you return to the neutral position. This exercise strengthens the muscles along your spine, aiding in maintaining a more upright posture.

By incorporating these posture correction exercises into your Wall Pilates routine, you'll target specific muscle groups that play a crucial role in supporting and improving your posture. Consistency is key, so make these exercises a regular part of your routine to experience lasting benefits for your overall alignment and posture.

Pelvic floor health through Pilates

Let's focus on an essential aspect of women's well-being – pelvic floor health. Wall Pilates offers targeted exercises to strengthen the pelvic floor muscles, promoting better control and overall health in this crucial area.

Pelvic Floor Contractions:
While standing or sitting, gently contract and lift the muscles around your pelvic floor. Imagine stopping the flow of urine midstream. Hold for a few seconds and then release. Repeat these contractions, gradually increasing the duration. This simple yet

effective exercise enhances awareness and strength in the pelvic floor muscles.

Bridge Pose Against the Wall:
Lie on your back with your feet against the wall and knees bent. Inhale as you lift your hips towards the ceiling, engaging your glutes and pelvic floor. Exhale as you lower back down. This controlled movement targets the pelvic floor while also strengthening the surrounding muscles.

Seated Leg Lifts with Wall Support:
Sit against the wall with your legs extended. Inhale as you lift one leg, engaging your pelvic floor muscles. Exhale as you lower it back down. Switch legs and repeat. This exercise combines core engagement with a focus on pelvic floor strength.

Incorporating these Pilates exercises into your routine contributes to pelvic floor health. The wall provides support, allowing you to concentrate on controlled movements that benefit this vital area. Consistency is key – make these exercises a regular part of your Wall Pilates practice for long-term pelvic floor well-being.

Modifications for different fitness levels

Addressing the diverse needs of individuals, Wall Pilates offers flexibility with modifications tailored for different fitness levels. Whether you're a beginner easing into a fitness routine or an experienced enthusiast seeking an extra challenge, these modifications ensure inclusivity.

Beginner Modifications:
- **Reduce the range of motion:** In exercises like leg lifts or wall push-ups, start with smaller movements to build strength gradually.
- **Increase rest intervals:** Allow more time between exercises to catch your breath and maintain control during each movement.
- **Use additional support:** If necessary, keep a chair nearby for balance or choose a closer wall to provide extra stability.

Intermediate Adjustments:
- **Gradually increase repetitions:** Progress from a comfortable number of repetitions to a slightly higher count as your endurance improves.
- **Add light resistance:** Incorporate small hand weights or resistance bands to intensify exercises without overwhelming your muscles.
- **Experiment with prop variations:** Challenge yourself by incorporating a Pilates ball or resistance

band to elevate the difficulty of specific movements.

Advanced Progressions:
- **Introduce complex movements:** Combine different exercises into flowing sequences to challenge coordination and control.
- **Reduce support from the wall:** For exercises like wall sits, gradually move farther away from the wall to increase the demand on your muscles.
- **Increase resistance:** Opt for heavier weights or stronger resistance bands to add intensity to upper and lower body exercises.

Remember, the key to effective modifications is to listen to your body. Tailor your Wall Pilates routine to match your current fitness level, gradually progressing as your strength and endurance improve. The wall remains a constant support, adapting to your needs and ensuring a personalized and rewarding fitness experience.

CHAPTER 5

Mind-Body Connection

Breathing techniques during Wall Pilates

The mind-body connection is a vital aspect of Wall Pilates, and mastering proper breathing techniques enhances the effectiveness of your workouts. Let's explore how intentional breathing can elevate your Pilates experience.

Diaphragmatic Breathing:
Begin by focusing on diaphragmatic breathing. Inhale deeply through your nose, allowing your diaphragm to expand and fill your lungs with air. Feel your abdomen rise. Exhale slowly through pursed lips, engaging your core as you release the breath. This rhythmic breathing creates a foundation for mindful movement.

Coordinated Breath with Movement:
Sync your breath with specific movements. For example, inhale during the preparatory phase of an exercise and exhale as you exert effort. During wall push-ups, inhale as you lower towards the wall and exhale as you push back. This coordination

enhances control, ensuring smoother and more controlled transitions.

Ribcage Expansion:

Visualize your ribcage expanding 360 degrees with each breath. As you inhale, feel your ribs expanding not just forward but also to the sides and back. This deep, expansive breath maximizes oxygen intake, promoting endurance and sustained energy during your Wall Pilates routine.

Breath Awareness in Rest Positions:

Pay attention to your breath during rest or recovery positions. Whether it's standing against the wall or taking a moment between exercises, maintain slow and controlled breathing. This conscious focus keeps you grounded and connected to the present moment.

By incorporating these breathing techniques, you cultivate a mindful approach to Wall Pilates. The breath becomes a guide, enhancing your awareness of movement and promoting a harmonious integration of the mind and body. As you embark on your Pilates journey, let your breath be the rhythm that propels you towards strength, flexibility, and holistic well-being.

Incorporating mindfulness into workouts

Embracing mindfulness is a transformative aspect of Wall Pilates, elevating your workout experience beyond mere physical exercise. Here's how you can weave mindfulness seamlessly into your routine:

Conscious Body Awareness:
Start by bringing your attention to each part of your body. As you engage in Wall Pilates exercises, focus on the sensations – the muscles contracting, the breath flowing, and the subtle shifts in posture. This heightened awareness creates a deeper connection between your mind and body.

Mindful Movement Sequences:
Rather than rushing through exercises, perform each movement with intention and deliberation. Visualize the muscles at work, notice your alignment, and feel the controlled transitions. This mindful approach not only enhances the effectiveness of the workout but also cultivates a sense of presence in the moment.

Positive Affirmations:
Incorporate positive affirmations into your Wall Pilates routine. As you perform each exercise, silently affirm your strength, resilience, and progress. Positive thoughts contribute to a more

uplifting and empowering workout experience, fostering a positive mindset.

Gratitude Practice:
Before or after your Wall Pilates session, take a moment to express gratitude for your body's capabilities. Acknowledge the effort you put into your workout and appreciate the support the wall provides. This practice instills a sense of gratitude that extends beyond the physical aspects of exercise.

Breath-Centered Mindfulness:
Build upon the breathing techniques mentioned earlier and center your mindfulness around your breath. Use each inhale and exhale as an anchor, grounding you in the present moment. The rhythmic flow of breath becomes a meditative element, calming the mind and enhancing focus.

By infusing mindfulness into your Wall Pilates routine, you create a holistic and enriching experience that extends beyond the physical benefits. Let your practice be a mindful journey, where each movement is an opportunity for self-discovery, growth, and a deeper connection with your overall well-being.

Stress relief and relaxation exercises

Incorporating stress relief and relaxation exercises into your Wall Pilates routine adds a valuable dimension to your overall well-being. Let's explore simple yet effective practices to unwind and find tranquility:

Wall-Assisted Deep Breathing:
Stand or sit comfortably with your back against the wall. Inhale deeply through your nose, letting your diaphragm expand. Exhale slowly through pursed lips. The wall provides support, allowing you to focus entirely on the calming rhythm of your breath. Repeat this deep breathing for several minutes to promote relaxation.

Legs Up the Wall Pose:
Lie on your back, placing your legs up against the wall. Rest your arms by your sides. This gentle inversion helps improve circulation and encourages a sense of calm. Close your eyes, focus on your breath, and let go of tension with each exhale. Hold this pose for 5-10 minutes as a soothing conclusion to your Wall Pilates session.

Mindful Stretching:
Engage in gentle stretches against the wall. Reach your arms overhead, feeling the lengthening of your

spine. Incorporate slow, deliberate movements, focusing on the sensations in your muscles. This mindful stretching not only promotes flexibility but also serves as a form of moving meditation, easing stress and tension.

Body Scan Meditation:
As you rest against the wall, perform a body scan meditation. Starting from your toes, mentally scan each part of your body, releasing any tension you encounter. Move gradually upwards, bringing awareness to each area. This meditation fosters relaxation and a heightened sense of body awareness.

Wall-Supported Savasana:
Conclude your Wall Pilates routine with a supported savasana against the wall. Lie on your back with your legs extended up the wall. Allow your arms to rest comfortably by your sides. Close your eyes and focus on your breath, letting go of any lingering tension. This restorative pose offers a serene conclusion to your practice.

By integrating these stress relief and relaxation exercises, you transform your Wall Pilates routine into a holistic and rejuvenating experience. The wall becomes a comforting backdrop, supporting not only your physical strength but also your mental and emotional well-being. Embrace these moments of tranquility, allowing them to be a sanctuary amidst the demands of daily life.

CHAPTER 6

Nutrition Tips for Women

Supporting Pilates workouts with a balanced diet

Fueling your body with a balanced diet is crucial to support your Wall Pilates workouts and optimize overall well-being. Here are practical nutrition tips for women engaging in this fitness routine:

1. Hydration is Key:
Ensure adequate hydration before, during, and after your workouts. Water plays a vital role in muscle function, joint lubrication, and overall energy levels. Aim for at least 8 cups of water daily, adjusting based on your activity level and individual needs.

2. Pre-Workout Nutrition:
Consume a balanced meal or snack 1-2 hours before your Wall Pilates session. Include a mix of carbohydrates and protein for sustained energy. Options like a banana with almond butter or Greek yogurt with berries provide a good balance to fuel your workout.

3. Post-Workout Recovery:

Optimize recovery with a post-workout meal or snack containing protein and carbohydrates. This helps replenish glycogen stores and supports muscle repair. A protein smoothie with fruits, or a chicken and vegetable wrap, are excellent choices for refueling after your Wall Pilates session.

4. Prioritize Protein:

Protein is essential for muscle repair and maintenance. Include lean protein sources such as chicken, fish, tofu, eggs, or legumes in your meals. Spread protein intake throughout the day to support sustained energy and muscle health.

5. Include Whole Foods:

Focus on whole, nutrient-dense foods. Incorporate a variety of colorful fruits, vegetables, whole grains, and healthy fats. These provide essential vitamins, minerals, and antioxidants to support overall health.

6. Portion Control:

Pay attention to portion sizes to avoid overeating. Listen to your body's hunger and fullness cues, and aim for balanced meals that include a mix of macronutrients.

7. Mindful Eating:

Practice mindful eating by savoring each bite and paying attention to hunger and fullness cues. Eating with awareness fosters a positive relationship with food and supports overall well-being.

8. Adequate Iron Intake:

Ensure sufficient iron intake, especially for women. Incorporate iron-rich foods like lean meats, beans, lentils, and dark leafy greens to support energy levels and prevent fatigue.

9. Consider Supplements:

If needed, consult with a healthcare professional to determine if supplements are necessary. Women, in particular, may require additional nutrients such as calcium, vitamin D, and omega-3 fatty acids.

By aligning your nutrition with your Wall Pilates routine, you provide your body with the essential nutrients needed for optimal performance, recovery, and overall health. It's about nourishing your body to enhance the benefits of your workouts and cultivate a balanced and sustainable lifestyle.

Hydration and its role in fitness

Hydration is a cornerstone of fitness, playing a vital role in supporting your Wall Pilates workouts and overall well-being. Let's explore the significance of hydration and practical tips to maintain optimal fluid balance:

1. Optimal Muscle Function:
Hydration is essential for proper muscle function. Dehydration can lead to muscle cramps, fatigue, and compromised performance during your Wall Pilates sessions. Ensuring adequate fluid intake supports muscle contraction, endurance, and overall strength.

2. Joint Lubrication:
Proper hydration aids in joint lubrication, reducing friction and supporting smooth movement during exercises. This is particularly beneficial in Wall Pilates, where controlled movements and joint flexibility are key components of the routine.

3. Temperature Regulation:
During exercise, your body temperature rises. Adequate hydration helps regulate body temperature through sweating. Staying hydrated ensures effective thermoregulation, preventing overheating and promoting a comfortable workout environment.

4. Energy Levels and Focus:
Dehydration can lead to feelings of fatigue, lethargy, and difficulty concentrating. Maintaining

optimal fluid balance supports sustained energy levels, allowing you to stay focused and engaged throughout your Wall Pilates routine.

5. Recovery and Nutrient Transport:

Hydration plays a role in post-workout recovery by facilitating nutrient transport to cells. Proper fluid balance aids in the delivery of essential nutrients to muscles, promoting efficient recovery and muscle repair after your Wall Pilates session.

Practical Hydration Tips:

- **Pre-Workout Hydration:** Drink water leading up to your workout to ensure you start well-hydrated.

- **During Exercise:** Sip water throughout your Wall Pilates session. While individual needs vary, a general guideline is to aim for about 7-10 ounces of water every 10-20 minutes during exercise.

- **Post-Workout Hydration:** Rehydrate after your workout to replenish fluid losses. Water is usually sufficient for moderate-intensity workouts, but for more prolonged or intense sessions, consider a sports drink that also replenishes electrolytes.

- **Monitor Urine Color:** Pay attention to the color of your urine. Pale yellow indicates good hydration, while dark yellow may signal dehydration.

- **Individualized Hydration:** Everyone's hydration needs are different. Factors such as climate, intensity of exercise, and individual physiology influence how much water you need. Listen to your body's cues and adjust your fluid intake accordingly.

Prioritizing hydration goes hand in hand with your Wall Pilates journey, ensuring that you perform at your best, recover effectively, and enjoy the holistic benefits of a well-hydrated body.

Recipes and meal plans for energy and recovery

Fueling your body with nutritious meals is essential for energy and recovery, especially when engaging in activities like Wall Pilates. Here are simple and balanced recipes along with a sample meal plan to support your fitness goals:

1. Energizing Breakfast:
Smoothie Bowl
- Ingredients
  - 1 cup mixed berries (strawberries, blueberries, raspberries)

- 1 banana
- 1/2 cup Greek yogurt
- 1 tablespoon chia seeds
- 1/4 cup granola
- Drizzle of honey
- Instructions:

1. Blend mixed berries, banana, and Greek yogurt until smooth.

2. Pour into a bowl and top with chia seeds, granola, and a drizzle of honey.

2. Nourishing Lunch:
Quinoa Salad with Grilled Chicken

- Ingredients:
  - 1 cup cooked quinoa
  - Grilled chicken breast, sliced
  - Mixed veggies (cherry tomatoes, cucumber, bell peppers)
  - Feta cheese
  - Olive oil and balsamic vinegar dressing
- Instructions:

1. Mix cooked quinoa with grilled chicken and veggies.

2. Top with crumbled feta cheese and drizzle with olive oil and balsamic vinegar.

3. Snack for Sustained Energy:
Apple Slices with Almond Butter

- Ingredients:

- 1 apple, sliced
  - 2 tablespoons almond butter
- Instructions:
   1. Spread almond butter on apple slices for a balanced and energy-boosting snack.

4. Recovery Dinner:
Salmon and Sweet Potato
- Ingredients:
  - Grilled salmon fillet
  - Baked sweet potato
  - Steamed broccoli
  - Lemon wedge
- Instructions:
   1. Grill salmon and serve with a baked sweet potato and steamed broccoli.
   2. Squeeze a lemon wedge for added flavor.

Sample Meal Plan:
Day 1:
- **Breakfast:** Smoothie Bowl
- **Lunch:** Quinoa Salad with Grilled Chicken
- **Snack:** Apple Slices with Almond Butter
- **Dinner:** Salmon and Sweet Potato

Day 2:
- **Breakfast:** Greek Yogurt Parfait with Berries and Granola

- **Lunch:** Turkey and Avocado Wrap with Whole Grain Tortilla
- **Snack:** Mixed Nuts and Dried Fruits
- **Dinner:** Vegetable Stir-Fry with Tofu and Brown Rice

Day 3:
- **Breakfast:** Oatmeal with Banana and Almond Milk
- **Lunch:** Chickpea Salad with Mixed Greens
- **Snack:** Cottage Cheese with Pineapple
- **Dinner:** Grilled Chicken Breast with Quinoa and Roasted Vegetables

Adjust portion sizes based on your individual needs and activity level. Stay hydrated throughout the day, and consider incorporating these recipes into your routine to support energy and recovery during and after your Wall Pilates workouts.

CHAPTER 7

Troubleshooting and Injury Prevention

Common mistakes to avoid

While engaging in Wall Pilates, it's essential to be aware of common mistakes to ensure a safe and effective workout. Let's highlight key errors to avoid, promoting injury prevention and overall well-being:

1. Poor Posture:
Avoid slouching or arching your back excessively. Maintain a neutral spine, especially when performing exercises against the wall. Proper posture ensures targeted muscle engagement and minimizes strain on your spine.

2. Overreliance on the Wall:
While the wall provides support, be mindful not to excessively rely on it. Use the wall as a guide for proper alignment, but aim to engage your core and stabilize yourself independently during exercises. This helps strengthen your muscles and improve overall stability.

3. Neglecting Warm-up:

Skipping a proper warm-up is a common mistake. Before diving into Wall Pilates exercises, take time for dynamic stretches and light cardio to increase blood flow and prepare your muscles for movement. Warming up reduces the risk of injury and enhances flexibility.

4. Incorrect Breathing Technique:

Pay attention to your breath. Avoid shallow breathing or holding your breath during exercises. Practice coordinated breathing, inhaling during the preparatory phase and exhaling during exertion. Proper breathing enhances oxygen flow to muscles and supports overall performance.

5. Ignoring Body Signals:

Listen to your body and avoid pushing through pain. If you experience discomfort beyond normal muscle fatigue, stop the exercise and reassess your form. Ignoring warning signals may lead to injury. It's okay to modify or skip an exercise if needed.

6. Lack of Variety:

Repeating the same set of exercises without variety can lead to muscle imbalances and boredom. Incorporate a diverse range of Wall Pilates movements to target different muscle groups and keep your routine engaging.

7. Poor Equipment Setup:
Ensure proper setup of any equipment used, such as a Pilates ball or resistance band. Check for wear and tear, and use equipment appropriate for your fitness level. Poor setup can compromise your safety and the effectiveness of the exercises.

8. Rushing Through Movements:
Maintain controlled and deliberate movements. Avoid rushing through exercises, as this diminishes their effectiveness and increases the risk of injury. Focus on quality over quantity, ensuring each movement is precise and controlled.

By being mindful of these common mistakes, you enhance your Wall Pilates experience, reduce the risk of injuries, and maximize the benefits of each session. Prioritize proper form, listen to your body, and make adjustments as needed for a safe and rewarding workout.

Tips for preventing injuries

Preventing injuries during your Wall Pilates workouts is paramount for a sustainable and enjoyable fitness journey. Here are practical tips to prioritize safety and minimize the risk of injuries:

1. Start with a Proper Warm-up:

Begin each session with a dynamic warm-up to increase blood flow and flexibility. Incorporate light cardio, dynamic stretches, and movements that mimic the exercises you'll be performing. A well-prepared body is more resilient to potential injuries.

2. Focus on Proper Form:
Maintain proper form throughout each exercise. Pay attention to your body alignment, engage your core, and ensure controlled movements. Proper form not only enhances the effectiveness of the exercise but also minimizes strain on joints and muscles.

3. Gradual Progression:
Avoid the temptation to progress too quickly. Gradually increase the intensity, duration, or complexity of your Wall Pilates routine. This allows your body to adapt to new challenges, reducing the risk of overuse injuries.

4. Listen to Your Body:
Be attentive to signals from your body. If you experience pain, discomfort, or unusual fatigue, take a break and reassess. Pushing through pain can lead to injuries. Modify or skip exercises if needed, and consult a healthcare professional if issues persist.

5. Hydration and Nutrition:

Stay adequately hydrated and maintain a balanced diet to support your body's energy levels and recovery. Proper nutrition contributes to muscle health and overall well-being, reducing the risk of fatigue-related injuries.

6. Include Rest Days:

Allow your body sufficient time to rest and recover. Incorporate rest days into your weekly routine to prevent overtraining. Rest is crucial for muscle repair and injury prevention.

7. Diversify Your Routine:

Include a variety of Wall Pilates exercises to target different muscle groups and movement patterns. This prevents muscle imbalances and reduces the risk of repetitive strain injuries. Mix up your routine to keep it engaging and challenging.

8. Use Proper Equipment:

Ensure that any equipment used, such as mats, Pilates balls, or resistance bands, is in good condition. Follow proper setup instructions and use equipment suitable for your fitness level. Poorly maintained or inappropriate equipment can pose safety risks.

9. Incorporate Recovery Practices:

Integrate recovery practices into your routine, such as stretching, foam rolling, or massage. These activities enhance flexibility, alleviate muscle tension, and contribute to injury prevention.

10. Seek Professional Guidance:
If you're new to Wall Pilates or have specific health concerns, consider seeking guidance from a certified Pilates instructor. They can provide personalized advice, correct your form, and tailor exercises to your individual needs.

By incorporating these injury prevention tips into your Wall Pilates routine, you create a foundation for a safe, effective, and sustainable fitness practice. Prioritize your well-being, listen to your body, and enjoy the transformative benefits of Pilates with reduced injury risk.

Listening to your body and adapting workouts

Listening to your body is a fundamental aspect of a safe and effective Wall Pilates practice. Here are key considerations and tips for tuning into your body's signals and adapting your workouts accordingly:

1. Sensation vs. Pain:

Distinguish between normal muscle fatigue and pain. Sensations of muscle engagement and challenge are expected, but sharp or persistent pain may indicate an issue. If you experience pain, stop the exercise, reassess your form, and consider modifying or skipping that particular movement.

2. Fatigue and Rest:

Acknowledge signs of fatigue and understand the importance of rest. If you're feeling overly tired or notice a decrease in your form, it's okay to take a break. Pushing through extreme fatigue can lead to compromised form and an increased risk of injury.

3. Modify When Needed:

Don't hesitate to modify exercises based on your current fitness level or any physical limitations. Whether it's adjusting the range of motion, using additional support, or choosing alternative movements, modifications allow you to tailor the workout to your individual needs.

4. Gradual Progression:

Listen to your body's response to progression. If you're introducing new exercises or increasing intensity, monitor how your body responds. Gradual progression allows for adaptation and reduces the risk of overuse injuries.

5. Be Mindful of Alignment:

Pay attention to your body's alignment during exercises. Proper alignment ensures effective engagement of targeted muscles and minimizes strain on joints. If you notice any deviations from proper form, make adjustments to maintain alignment.

6. Stay Hydrated:

Dehydration can impact your performance and increase the risk of fatigue-related injuries. Listen to your body's thirst signals and ensure you stay adequately hydrated before, during, and after your Wall Pilates session.

7. Respect Individual Limits:

Every individual has different fitness levels and capabilities. It's crucial to respect your own limits and not compare yourself to others. Focus on your progress and listen to what your body is telling you on any given day.

8. Recovery Practices:

Incorporate recovery practices into your routine. Stretching, foam rolling, and gentle mobility exercises can aid in muscle recovery and flexibility. These practices also provide an opportunity to check in with your body and identify any areas of tightness or discomfort.

9. Consult Professionals:

If you have specific health concerns or are new to Wall Pilates, consider consulting with a certified Pilates instructor or healthcare professional. They can offer guidance on proper form, suggest modifications, and ensure that your workout aligns with your individual needs.

By cultivating a mindful awareness of your body's signals and being responsive to its needs, you enhance the safety and effectiveness of your Wall Pilates workouts. Listen, adapt, and celebrate the journey towards improved strength, flexibility, and overall well-being.

Conclusion

Recap of key takeaways

In conclusion, our exploration of Wall Pilates for women has been a journey of discovery and empowerment. Let's recap the key takeaways that encapsulate the essence of this fitness approach:

1. Accessible and Effective:
Wall Pilates provides a practical and accessible way for women to engage in effective workouts. The support of the wall offers stability, making it suitable for various fitness levels and addressing diverse wellness goals.

2. Holistic Benefits:
Beyond physical fitness, Wall Pilates fosters a holistic approach to well-being. From building core strength and improving posture to cultivating a mindful mind-body connection, the benefits extend beyond the workout, positively impacting daily life.

3. Mindfulness Matters:
The incorporation of breathing techniques and mindfulness elevates Wall Pilates to more than just a physical exercise. It becomes a moment of connection with oneself, fostering a sense of calm and mental clarity amidst life's demands.

4. Individualized Progression:

The gradual progression inherent in Wall Pilates allows women to tailor their workouts to individual needs. Whether addressing core weakness, posture concerns, or overall fitness, the adaptable nature of these exercises supports sustainable progress.

5. Real-Life Transformations:

The real-life success stories and before-and-after transformations illustrate the tangible impact of Wall Pilates on women's lives. From building strength and confidence to overcoming challenges, these stories inspire and resonate with the transformative potential of this fitness approach.

6. Injury Prevention and Adaptability:

Prioritizing proper form, listening to one's body, and adapting workouts are crucial for injury prevention. Wall Pilates empowers women to embrace a mindful and adaptive approach, ensuring a safe and effective fitness journey.

7. Motivation in Consistency and Progress:

Motivational anecdotes highlight the importance of consistency, inner strength, and the uplifting power of progress. Small, consistent efforts with the wall can lead to significant positive changes, both physically and emotionally.

In embracing Wall Pilates, women embark on a journey that goes beyond exercise – it's about self-discovery, empowerment, and a mindful connection with the body. As we conclude this exploration, may each woman find strength, resilience, and joy in her unique Wall Pilates journey. Here's to a future filled with holistic well-being and the ongoing pursuit of a healthier, happier life.

Encouragement for continued Wall Pilates practice

As you conclude this exploration into the world of Wall Pilates, I want to leave you with words of encouragement for your continued practice. Remember, your journey with the wall is a personal and empowering one, and every effort contributes to your well-being.

Consistency is Key:
In the realm of Wall Pilates, consistency is your greatest ally. Small, regular sessions with the wall add up over time, creating a foundation of strength, flexibility, and resilience. Trust the process, and let each engagement with the wall be a step forward on your journey.

Celebrate Progress, Big or Small:
Take a moment to acknowledge and celebrate your progress. Whether it's mastering a challenging exercise, feeling increased flexibility, or experiencing enhanced well-being, every achievement, no matter how small, is a victory. Recognize your efforts and embrace the positive changes you're cultivating.

Listen to Your Body's Wisdom:
Your body communicates with you, offering cues and insights. Listen attentively during your Wall Pilates practice. If something feels right, embrace it. If you need a moment to rest or modify an exercise, honor that intuition. Your body's wisdom guides your practice and contributes to a sustainable, enjoyable journey.

Embrace Adaptability:
Life is dynamic, and so is your Wall Pilates practice. Embrace adaptability in your routine. If time is limited, opt for a shorter session. If you're feeling particularly energized, challenge yourself with a variety of exercises. The versatility of Wall Pilates allows you to tailor your practice to your current needs.

Make it Your Sanctuary:

View your time with the wall as a sanctuary—a moment for self-care, rejuvenation, and connection. Whether it's a brief session or a more extended workout, let it be a space where you nourish your body, mind, and spirit. The wall becomes your steadfast companion on this journey of holistic well-being.

Encourage Others Along the Way:
If you've experienced the transformative power of Wall Pilates, consider sharing your journey with others. Your encouragement might inspire someone else to embark on their own path to wellness. A supportive community can be a powerful motivator and source of inspiration.

As you continue your Wall Pilates practice, may each session be a step towards greater vitality, joy, and self-discovery. The wall is not just a support; it's a canvas for your unique journey to unfold. Keep moving, keep embracing the journey, and may your relationship with the wall be a source of continual growth and empowerment.

www.ingramcontent.com/pod-product-compliance
Lightning Source LLC
Chambersburg PA
CBHW060841260726
48661CB00002B/536